Survivor's Guide to Chemo

Information, Suggestions and Tips from a Cancer Survivor

By Deborah Waun, MA, LPC, BCPCC

Foreword by nationally renowned gynecologic oncologist
John L. Powell, M.D., FACOG, FACS

PublishAmerica
Baltimore

First printing

PublishAmerica has allowed this work to remain exactly as the author intended, verbatim, without editorial input.

ISBN: 1-60813-089-4
PUBLISHED BY PUBLISHAMERICA, LLLP
www.publishamerica.com
Baltimore

Printed in the United States of America

Dedication

This book is dedicated to my wonderful mother (Alison Waun) who has spent her entire life helping others (as a mother, as a pastor's wife, as a caseworker for social services and as a DAR member helping the community). She has set an example for other Christian women to follow. God gave me one of the greatest blessings there is by allowing me to have her as my mother. She sacrificed things for herself so she could give more to me; she sacrificed time for herself by working to help provide for me, and then giving me what little leisure time she had; and she continues to give of herself in whatever way she can in order to give me a better life. I am here today because my loving mother nursed me back to health, went with me to every doctor's appointment and chemo treatment, and encouraged me every step of the way.

Special Thanks

To my heroes: Dr. John L. Powell and Dr. Adnan Taj-Eldin for saving my life.

To my best friends: Mary Hughes and Laurel Schaefer for their prayers, cards, phone calls and encouragement.

To my brother: the Rev. Dr. William G. Waun for coming to my rescue whenever I needed him.

To all the nurses at the Zimmer Center and New Hanover Regional Medical Center who helped me through the surgery and chemo treatments.

And to all my friends and family who prayed for me, emailed me, sent flowers and cards, and called to support me.

Contents

Foreword

I have been treating women with ovarian cancer for over thirty years. Many changes have occurred in that time period in surgical techniques, new chemotherapy drugs, anti-emetics, and bone-marrow stimulating medicines. Throughout those years I have always been amazed by and admired the courage, strength, determination to survive and endure, gratitude, and kindness of my patients. Deborah Waun's book will be a helpful guide with useful tips, and inspiration to other women facing the challenge of ovarian cancer.

The fortunate person, in my opinion, is he/she to whom the gods have granted the power either to do something which is worth recording or to write what is worth reading, and most fortunate of all is the person who can do both.

John L. Powell, M.D., FACOG, FACS
Director, Gynecologic Oncology
New Hanover Regional Medical Center
Southeastern Area Health Education Center
Professor Obstetrics and Gynecology
University of North Carolina School of Medicine

Introduction

This is a straightforward handbook with the facts about making it through chemo treatments with as little pain and discomfort as possible. These ideas and tips are taken from my personal experience. I wish I had a book like this to refer to when I had questions because I have included brand name products to have on hand and specific things you can do to help relieve the pain. My desire to help you inspired me to write this book. I have written this in such a way so that you can just go straight to the tips and suggestions to get immediate help or you can read on about my experiences. I did this because sometimes you may not feel like reading and hunting through a book to find what you need. The tips are bolded, bulleted and the first thing you will read in each section. I have started this book with some background about myself and my personal experience finding out I had cancer, making it through surgery and struggling to survive. Knowledge is power.

I guess everyone must have the same reaction… "No, not me!" I was 48 and had been very healthy all of my life so the idea of cancer was out of the question.

I am a preacher's daughter who grew up in a small town in Indiana. I am the only girl and the baby of the family so I got lots of attention growing up. I led a relatively normal life and moved to California when I was 27. I lived there for 14 years where I worked in the entertainment industry. In 2000, I moved to Georgia to help take care of my father who had been diagnosed with an incurable rare illness. I helped my mother care for him for the last 6 months of his life. At the time, I believed that would be the hardest thing I ever had to do but life is full of surprises.

I enjoyed living in California and especially loved my job in casting. It was fun being able to find the right actor for the part. However, casting can also be very stressful at times. And stress breaks down the immune system. I was fortunate to grow up in a Christian home with loving parents who did everything to help me have a good life. So when my dad got sick I knew it was time to make some changes and help him. I quit my job in casting and moved to Atlanta to live with my parents and help care for my father. This was a very difficult time because I watched my big strong dad deteriorate and become weak and helpless. My dad had been a preacher all of his life. He dedicated his life to serving the Lord and helping to lead others to Christ. I spent my life watching my dad lead and direct. He was a force and everyone knew it. Now he was so weak he couldn't get out of bed. My security disappeared before my eyes. Even though I was an adult in my 40's, I still felt like a little girl when I lost him. On December 16, 2001, I was with him when he passed away. It was during that time that I decided I wanted to help people who were going through rough times. While working full time, I pursued my Master's degree in Psychology and I am currently a Licensed Professional Counselor.

I continued living with my mother in Georgia while I completed the required supervision for licensure. In the meantime, my brother and his family moved to North Carolina and we began thinking about how nice it would be to live near family but still stay in a warm climate. Once we made the decision to move, things started happening quickly. My mother and I did all of the packing for the move ourselves. My mother was 80 so I tried to do most of it. I took on everything. I contacted realtors, researched new homes in North Carolina on the internet, dealt with our financial advisors, screened moving companies and packed every day for 2 ½ months. When the movers came, I helped them carry things to the moving van. I cleaned the house and packed the car. I drove us 9 hours to our new home. Then I helped the movers unload the moving van. I never stopped. I went through all the boxes in our garage (which was stacked full of boxes). I unpacked, moved furniture and organized the heavy boxes by moving them to certain areas in the garage. This was all done in July and August in the south when the temperatures were in the 90's. At the same time I was filling out insurance paperwork for damaged property from the move, working on getting my counseling license in North Carolina, and looking for a job. My brother and sister-in-law warned me to slow down and even take a vacation but not me! There was work to be done! I say all of this as a warning to others. We don't know what causes cancer but we do know that stress weakens the immune system.

In mid August I started feeling sick. It began by feeling like I couldn't burp or pass gas. Then my stomach and abdomen became bloated. I also had a fever. The fever started at 103 degrees for one night but after that it ranged between 99 and 101 degrees. My stomach began cramping and I lost my appetite. I began feeling sick all of the time and didn't eat much. Looking back, I realize I had other symptoms that I chalked up to getting older. Five months prior to getting sick, my abdomen started to bloat and I had acid reflux when I went to bed. I was also on edge and irritable much of the time. And I had to urinate more frequently.

Since I had just moved to North Carolina, I did not have a doctor. My brother who already lived here was in the Navy and therefore had a Navy physician and couldn't recommend a doctor.

So I went to the Urgent Care where a doctor examined me and took blood and urine tests. The tests did not indicate any problem and my white blood cell count was not elevated. Since my white blood cells were in the normal range, I thought it must not be cancer. I assumed that if I had cancer, my white blood cells would be fighting off the infection and I would therefore have an elevated white blood count. I now know that you cannot rely on that. The Urgent Care doctor's diagnosis was gastroenteritis and he suggested that I see a Gastroenterologist. He prescribed an elixir (Belladonna®) to help with the stomach cramps. I immediately made an appointment with a Gastroenterologist but his first opening was not until October 12th and this was mid August. There are only two Gastroenterologists in Jacksonville, NC and they were both booked solid until that time. My next development was diarrhea. As I mentioned before, I lost my appetite since my stomach always hurt. I felt sick all of the time and I was losing weight. Since I was not getting better, I went to the Emergency Room at the local hospital. I waited for 6 hours before I saw a doctor. That doctor examined me, took more blood and urine tests and an x-ray. All tests came back clean because they were not testing or looking for cancer. This doctor agreed that it must be gastroenteritis and sent me home. I suffered for 6 long weeks while I continued to wait for my appointment with the Gastroenterologist. Think of how bad you feel when you have the stomach flu for a day or two. Now multiply that by 45 days. I was desperate to find out what was happening to me. I researched the internet with my symptoms trying to figure out what was wrong. One possibility I came up with was parasites. I went back to the Urgent Care and asked them to take a stool sample and test for parasites. While I was there the doctor said he would pull some strings and get me in with a local MD in a few days. This was a big turning point. When I went to see the MD, (Dr. Eldin), he examined me and felt a tumor (a big tumor). I still wonder how 3 other doctors did not feel that tumor when I was examined before. If you know that something is wrong with you, be persistent and find a doctor who can help you. Don't wait! Who knows what stage I would have been in if I had just continued to wait to see the gastroenterologist. Two days later on September 25th I had a CT scan which revealed a huge tumor in my abdomen. This information was immediately given to Dr. Eldin who called me into his office right away. He explained to me that I had a very large tumor (basketball sized) in my abdomen but it might not be cancer. He suggested that I see a cancer specialist at the Zimmer Center in Wilmington (1 ½ hours away). I was sick and scared and asked him to please call the specialist and try to get me in right away. He did not ask a nurse to call, he immediately made the call. When he left the room to call the specialist, I prayed that God would help me and that the specialist would see me right away. When Dr. Eldin came back he said that the specialist would see me the next day at 9:00 am. What are the chances that a busy well-known cancer specialist (Dr. John L. Powell) would be available to see me first thing the next day? As it turned out, Dr. Powell is not only well-known but he is one of the nation's leading gynecologic oncologists. I was too sick to drive and my mother was 80 with vision problems. Plus neither of us knew our way to or around Wilmington. We called my brother (the Rev. Dr. William G. Waun) who dropped everything and changed his schedule to take us. Since I knew I had a tumor I packed a bag on the off-chance that they would admit me. We also took the CT scan with us. Dr. John Powell met with us, looked at the CT scan and didn't pull any punches. He looked me in the eye and told me I had a very large tumor that was ovarian cancer. He said I needed surgery including a complete hysterectomy, removal of my appendix, lymph nodes and omentum. My head was reeling. I was shocked. This couldn't be true. I questioned Dr. Powell asking him if it couldn't possibly be benign. The answer was a quick and certain "No." What does this mean? What is my prognosis? The answer was that we would have to wait until the surgery. I was ushered to another room where I was examined and several vials of blood were drawn. The realization of everything was setting in and a wave of fear and sorrow overwhelmed me. I cried and thought about my life and how I hadn't accomplished much. I was worried that I might not survive the surgery. One of Dr. Powell's nurses (Nicole) came in and reassured me that I would make it through the surgery and things might not be as bad as I was thinking. Knowing that I needed it, I felt an urgency to get it over. I knew Dr. Powell would have a full surgery schedule and I was concerned that I would have to wait several days or longer. I prayed that he would work me in right away. When I asked him when he could perform the surgery, he said he would check his schedule and try to work me in the next day. I believe this was another answer to prayer. The surgery was set for noon the next day at New Hanover Regional Medical Center which is adjacent to the Zimmer Center. My mother and brother were waiting for me in another room. We were reunited and then we all proceeded down the hall to the hospital and to the room where I would be spending the next week. My mother and brother stayed with me until I was settled in and then they headed back to Jacksonville. That's when the fear really set in. There I was all alone in my hospital room with all my thoughts and fears crashing in on me.

When you are facing major surgery and you know you have cancer, the worst scenarios flood your mind. I lay in my hospital bed praying and quietly crying when the sweetest nurse came in. Her name was Shirley and she asked me what she could do to help. I asked her if she would pray for me. She did not hesitate. She hugged me and then took my hand and prayed for me. Then she sat with me and reassured me that everything would be okay. She was there when I needed someone. I had several attentive nurses and very good care during my hospital stay.

The next day before the surgery, (thanks to Shirley), several nurses came into my room. We formed a circle holding hands and they all prayed for me. This was a great comfort to me. My mother, brother and sister-in-law were also there. Before I knew it they were wheeling me down for surgery. My family was taken to a waiting room. I was taken to the pre-op area where I met the Assisting Doctor, the Anesthesiologist and the Operating Room Nurse. Her name was Ruth. I remember how kind Ruth was. She promised she would watch over me during the surgery and she explained about my option to have a shot for pain given at the base of the spine. I am glad that I elected to have that shot because I don't remember even getting it. The last thing I remember was my conversation with Ruth. The next thing I remember is waking up in my hospital room with a tube down my throat.

The surgery had included a complete hysterectomy, removal of my lymph nodes, appendix and omentum. Dr. Powell told me that he always removes those body parts during surgery because that is where the cancer cells like to hide. The next evening, after my surgery, my hero (Dr. Powell) came in with good news. I call Dr. Powell "my hero" because he saved my life. What is the definition of a hero? Webster's dictionary defines hero as, "one distinguished for action, a brave man, noble, conqueror, champion, man of great courage, a man among men." I submit that doctors who dedicate themselves to trying to save lives and go into battle daily against disease are heroes. They have to face people everyday with bad news and sometimes watch them get worse while they do their best to fight their illness. I couldn't help myself but my hero stepped in and saved me. I can't think of anyone who better fits the definition of hero than Dr. Powell. I was still on a lot of medication so I did not understand everything Dr. Powell told me at the time. I got some things confused and mixed up. Doctors always have a way of showing up in your hospital room after your family has left or before they have arrived. Your family can sit there in your hospital room with you all day and as soon as they leave, the doctor magically shows up. Anyway, he told me that I was in Stage One (which is the best stage). He said that he believes he got all of the cancer and all of my organs looked clean. This was all wonderful news. Somehow I did not hear all of that. It was a few days before I understood that things were really looking up. However, Dr. Powell recommended that I begin chemo in a month just in case there were any hidden cancer cells that he could not see.

I was fortunate to have a private room and wonderful nurses. Since visiting hours were over by the time I woke up, my family had left. But I wasn't alone for long. I had caring nurses checking on me all night. I also had several phone calls from friends and family. Three things I advise anyone to take to the hospital if they are having surgery are ear plugs, a neck pillow and an eye mask. The ear plugs muffled all the hospital noises, the neck pillow really helped me sleep since I could only lie on my back, and the eye mask helped because there was always a light on in my room.

I was in the hospital for seven days after surgery where I was on a liquid diet most of the time. They switched me to solid food the morning that I was released to go home but nothing appealed to me. I ate 3 tiny bites of a biscuit but just couldn't bring myself to eat anything else. Before I knew it, my mother and brother were there to take me home. This was October 3rd. I was very weak and still did not feel good but I was anxious to go home. My brother was so kind to come and get me 1 ½ hours there and back and he made me as comfortable as possible in the back seat of his minivan. My mother brought a blanket for me which was a great idea because it took me a long time to get my body temperature regulated. I was always cold. When I got home I was greeted by my sweet little parrot Bo who showed how much she missed me by kissing and kissing my fingers over and over. I was fortunate that my mother took care of her while I was in the hospital.

Before I left the hospital I was told I could eat anything. BIG MISTAKE! I decided to have a banana and some crackers (Saltines) for my meal. I found out later that the banana was the worst thing I could have eaten because it is hard to digest. And I found out the hard way. It hit me around midnight and lasted for several hours. The pain was terrible. It felt like my stomach and intestines were on fire. All I could do was stand and pace while holding my stomach and crying. At the time I did not realize it was the banana. I was worried that something serious was wrong. The next day I felt better but still felt sick. I called the doctor's office and spoke to his nurse (Debbie) who told me it was most likely the banana. She suggested that I take Maalox to soothe my stomach and it really helped. She also prescribed some medication (Aciphex®) which helps break down the acid in the stomach. In addition, she suggested that I try eating Jell-O, popsicles, or pudding along with drinking Special K water, Pedialyte or Gatorade. These are all foods/fluids that are easy to digest along with helping to keep you hydrated and provide nutrients. I called Debbie several times with questions while I was recuperating and she was always very kind and helpful.

One thing to be aware of is that you do not need to get your prescriptions fully filled. You can get them half-filled until you see if you need more. I spent a lot of money getting a pain medication (Oxycodone®) filled only to find out that I didn't need it.

I experienced pain in my shoulders, upper back and sides which I think was trapped gas. My mother suggested putting heat on the area where I had the pain. I couldn't see how heat could help but much to my surprise the pain went away! So every time I had that type of pain, I heated up a little microwavable bean bag and held it to the area of pain and after a while the pain was gone.

On October 8th (5 days after being released from the hospital and 11 days after surgery) I had my staples removed. I have a large incision starting approximately 2" below my breasts down to my pelvis. There were a lot of staples to remove. The staples are removed with what looks like a large staple remover. They come out easily but it really stings. The worst part was when they removed the staples by my naval! Ouch! Dr. Powell said I was healing well and asked if I had any questions before starting chemo. By this time I knew enough (thanks to my sister-in-law, Cynthia, for doing the research) to ask what stage I was in and what my CA-125 count was. He said I was in stage 1C. My CA-125 count was 126 and needs to be below 30. He said he got all the cancer and my appendix and other organs all looked clean. He gave me a good prognosis and said I had a 90% chance of full recovery. My family and I prayed and thanked God for the good prognosis. Dr. Powell then advised that I have the chemo therapy to ensure that any hidden cancer cells would be destroyed. He said I would be scheduled for 6 hours of chemo once a month for 6 months beginning November 5th. Then he gave me a carrying bag full of literature. While I was relieved and grateful for the good prognosis, at the same time, I was filled with dread over having to take chemo.

My mother was caring for me at home and would leave to run short errands during the day. The next day after having my staples removed, I was standing in the kitchen when I felt water running down my leg. I couldn't understand what was happening. I rushed to the bathroom where I continued to release water. It felt as though I had no control over my bladder and the color was pink which led me to believe there was blood in it. I was home alone and I began to panic. I called the doctor's office in Wilmington but had to leave a message and wait for them to call back. I tried calling my mother on her cell phone but it went straight to voice mail. I remembered that my brother (who lives right down the street) was home until noon that day so I called him. I didn't know what was happening to me and I was scared to be alone. My brother came right over and stayed with me until my mother got home. The nurse returned my call and explained that it could be two things. It could be a bladder infection or it could be that some stitches around my vagina had dissolved which had been holding back some fluid. She prescribed an antibiotic in case it was a bladder infection and told me to go see my local MD for a urine test. It turned out that in my case it was both of the scenarios. After one day everything cleared up, but at the time, it was quite a scare.

Having a hysterectomy is major surgery and it takes a long time to fully recover. Not to mention that I was malnourished and dehydrated due to not eating anything except crackers for six weeks prior to the surgery. I was very weak and even had difficulty walking at first. I did not have an appetite and nothing sounded good. Dr. Powell warned me that I needed protein to build up my white blood cell count but I could not bring myself to eat meat. It took a couple of months but I slowly regained my appetite. My education has taught me that sometimes you have to start by retraining your brain, so I started watching the *Food Network* and my mother made me homemade soups and stews. I began by just eating the broth and gravy and worked my way up to eating the vegetables and finally, after a couple of months, the meat.

I don't know why I had to go through this experience but I know that it has made me more sympathetic to people who are ill. At one point, I felt so sick and the pain was so bad that I actually thought that death might not be so bad. I had never had a thought like that before in my life. Now I understand how people who are in pain and have a terminal illness might not want to live. I want to use my experience to help others going through similar situations.

On November 5, 2007, I started my first chemo treatment at the Zimmer Center. It was an all-day process and I spent 6 hours in the chemo chair. While I mention certain things that happened to me during the time I was taking chemo, this is not to say that those things will happen to you. Everyone is different. All in all, the chemo was not as bad as I had expected and the chemo nurses took excellent care of me. I was never left alone and they took a personal interest in my comfort every time I received a treatment. The following chapters are filled with information based on my experience and what I learned during my fight for survival.

Tips and Suggestions

Familiarize Yourself with Your Treatment Plan and Possible Side Effects

When your cancer is first diagnosed, your doctor will review a treatment plan with you. This may involve surgery, radiation therapy, chemotherapy, hormone therapy, and biologic immunotherapy or some combination of those treatments.

All of these regimes kill cells. In the process of killing the cancer cells, some healthy cells are also destroyed. That is what causes the side effects of the cancer treatments. You may experience any or none of the following:

- Sore mouth or throat or dry mouth
- Sores or white patches on your lips, mouth or throat
- Loss of appetite
- A change in sense of taste or smell
- Weight loss or weight gain
- Lactose intolerance
- Diarrhea
- Vomiting and nausea
- Stomach pain
- Constipation

- Pain or burning when you urinate
- Frequent urination
- Not being able to urinate
- Reddish or bloody urine
- Dental problems
- Fatigue
- Depression
- Aching in the bones
- Muscle, bone, or joint pain
- Weak, sore or achy muscles
- Rectal bleeding
- Shaking or trembling
- Hearing loss
- Itching or hives
- Severe skin rash
- Darkened, yellow, brittle or cracked nails
- Warmth or redness in your face, neck, arms or upper chest
- Swelling in your face or hands
- Swelling or tingling in your mouth or throat
- Tingling/numbing/burning sensation in your hands, arms, legs or feet
- Chest tightness
- Fast, slow, or uneven heartbeat
- Light-headedness or fainting
- Trouble breathing
- Bloody or black, tarry stools
- Changes in vision
- Fever, chills, or cough
- Ringing in your ears or trouble hearing
- Unusual bleeding, bruising or weakness
- Hair loss
- Anemia

- Confusion or memory loss
- Loss of balance or clumsiness
- Walking problems
- Jaw pain
- Onset of menopause/hormonal changes which may include hot flashes
- Infertility
- Earaches
- Headaches
- Impotence (for men)

Please note that some people don't experience any side effects. Everyone is different and many things factor into whether or not you will have side effects. These factors include the type of cancer you have, the part of your body being treated, the type and length of treatment, the dose of treatment, your diet, your personal outlook or attitude and the medications you are taking to prevent side effects. There are lots of medications being prescribed that can prevent almost any side effect out there. I experienced loss of appetite, weight loss, some lactose intolerance, some constipation, some fatigue (although not as bad as most), one bout of rectal bleeding due to eating popcorn, a one time experience of numbness & tingling in my hands, arms, legs and feet, a one time experience of feeling nauseous, hair loss and aching in my bones. The worst of the side effects for me was the aching. This may have been due partly to the chemo but it is mostly attributed to a side effect of a shot (Neulasta®) I had to take after each chemo treatment to increase my white blood cells. This shot caused terrible aching in my back, legs and feet. The aching usually lasted around 4 days. Generally, side effects disappear after your treatments stop.

It's Not Only Okay but It Is Necessary to Eat High Calorie Foods

My doctor and a nutritionist at the Zimmer Center recommended higher calorie foods with lots of protein. Dairy products such as milk and cheese are great unless you are lactose intolerant. Forget the diet foods and sugar-free foods. This is the time to build up your body so you can withstand the effects of the cancer and the treatments. You may not feel like eating a lot so make a point to eat foods that are higher in calories. Some higher calorie food suggestions (that are not spicy) include: pancakes, cinnamon buns, doughnuts, cheeseburgers (but not from fast-food restaurants), grilled cheese sandwiches, milk-based soups, potato salad, biscuits, most meat, ice cream, milkshakes, cake, pie, and cookies.

There Are Many Reasons Why You May Lose Your Appetite

Most people lose their appetite at some point during the duration of their chemo treatments. However, some people actually gain weight. While most women do not like to think about gaining weight, it can be a good thing when you are taking chemo. You may lose your appetite due to the chemo treatments, due to the cancer or due to your anxiety. Everyone reacts differently. I am a licensed professional counselor and have seen people lose their appetite due to fear, anxiety and depression. All of these emotions are normal when you are battling cancer. You may also experience a change in taste or smell which can influence your appetite. I was sick for 6 weeks prior to having surgery to remove a large ovarian tumor. During that time, I lost my appetite because I was experiencing stomach pain and diarrhea. After surgery, I still did not have an appetite and my stomach was very sensitive. I explained some of this in the introduction of the book so I won't go into detail again. My doctor prescribed two medications for me. One was supposed to help in the digestion process (Aciphex® in pill form) and the other one was to increase my appetite (Megestrol Acetate® in liquid form). I have to confess that I only took one dose of Megestrol

Acetate® because I hated the taste. The way I regained my appetite was by watching the *Food Network* and giving myself time to heal. Even my favorite foods like bread and chocolate did not appeal to me and the thought of meat was disgusting! I knew I needed to eat meat because I needed the protein to build up my white blood cells. I started by eating homemade chicken and beef soups. I only ate the broth at first and then I ate some vegetables. Next I ate some homemade beef stew. Once again, I only ate the gravy and vegetables. I kept watching food programs and pretty soon the food started looking good. The next thing I tried was Chef Boyardee Beef Ravioli. I used to eat it when I was a kid and it appealed to me again. The ravioli has some processed meat in it which may not be the healthiest thing to eat but it got me started eating meat again. Not long after that I began to eat the meat in the stew. I continued to watch food programs and slowly regained my appetite. I am a big believer in Cognitive Behavior therapy. First you must change your thinking (cognitive) and then your behavior will follow. Some other ideas that may help you with your appetite include:

- Have foods on hand that appealed to you when you were a child
- Keep snacks on hand. I began with Cheez-Its.
- Remember that you can get protein from other sources like peanut butter
- Liquid meals are an option such as Ensure
- Sometimes cold food is more appealing like pudding, yogurt or popsicles
- Exercise stimulates appetite

If You Are Experiencing Nausea, Talk to Your Doctor

There are many different medications that can help you with nausea. My doctor prescribed three different medications. Dexamethasone® which is a steroid that helps prevent nausea; and Ondansetron®) which works on both the peripheral and central nerves. It reduces the activity of the vagus nerve, which activates the vomiting center in the medulla oblongata (the lower portion of the brain stem) and serotonin receptors. These were given to me in an IV prior to each chemo treatment and in a pill form. I was told to take 5 tablets of Dexamethasone® at 10:00 the night before taking chemo and 5 more tablets at 6:00 the morning of my chemo treatment. I was also prescribed to take 1 tablet of Ondansetron® at bedtime on the night of my chemo treatment and continue taking it twice a day for three days after my chemo treatment. In addition, Prochlorperazine® was prescribed to be used as needed when I felt nauseated after chemo treatments. It acts by blocking dopamine receptors. Basically, the brain has neurotransmitters that send messages to your stomach which can cause the nauseated feeling. Prochlorperazine® blocked those messages and really worked for me. I only felt nauseated once a few days after my first chemo treatment. It was a horrible feeling because it was combined with other side effects such as breaking out in a cold sweat, feeling dizzy, having severe tingling like getting an electric shock in my whole body and a lot of pressure in my ears. At the first sign of feeling sick, I took Prochlorperazine® and about ½ hour later, I felt better. However, if your medications are not working for you, tell your doctor and try the same things you would do if you had the stomach flu. Try eating crackers, toast, ice chips, carbonated drinks like ginger ale, yogurt, or rice. Sometimes sucking on a mint candy will help. Other techniques you may want to try include breathing deeply and slowly when you feel nauseated and using relaxation therapy.

When You Start to Feel Sorry for Yourself (and You Will), It Is Okay to Cry

Crying is a way to release your emotions and it can be a good thing to do as long as you do not wallow in your sorrows. I had times when I really felt sorry for myself. I felt helpless and I questioned God. I couldn't understand why this was happening to me. I allowed myself some time to be sad but I reminded myself that there are others who had it much worse than I. I started thinking of ways that I might be able to help others who were going through what I was. I also started counting my blessings. Every time I thought of something negative (like not having a husband to help me), I thought of a positive (I had my mother). When I thought about all the medical bills that were piling up and how I did not have a job, I thought about how nice it was to not have to worry about trying to take care of myself and still have to work. When you are told that you have cancer, the world stops spinning for a moment. Time just stands still as you are hit in the face with something you just cannot believe. Cancer is something that happens to other people, not me! I have been healthy all of my life. This cannot be true! But when the doctor looks you in the eye and tells you it is true beyond a shadow of a doubt, you are slapped in the face by reality. The next thing I felt was hopelessness. I have cancer so my life must be over. At the time that I was diagnosed, the doctor did not know my prognosis because he was making his diagnosis based upon a CT scan and my symptoms. He would not know how advanced the cancer was until surgery. He took a blood sample and they ran a test called CA-125 which is an indicator for cancer but they did not have the results until later. In my case, the CT scan showed that I had a tumor the size of a basketball. It was not shaped like a basketball or everyone would have known that I had a tumor. It was elongated and hidden in my abdomen. The doctor I saw (Dr. Powell) is a full professor at UNC-Chapel Hill and one of the nation's leading gynecologic oncologists so he knew (based on his experience) that it was ovarian cancer. The night in the hospital before my surgery was very scary. I did not know what to expect (i.e., how bad the cancer was, if it had spread, or even if I would survive the surgery). All of those thoughts kept swirling through my head. My mother and brother stayed with me in my hospital room as long as they were allowed but after they left, I was left alone with those thoughts. This was the worst night of my life. I admit that I cried a lot that night. I cried out of fear and sorrow for myself. We all have our moments of weakness. It is part of being human.

Don't Eat Popcorn

I had a bad experience which has been attributed to eating popcorn the day before getting one of my chemo treatments. I thought eating popcorn would be a good source of roughage which would help with digestion. Boy, was I wrong! The popcorn seemed to gather in my intestines where it hardened. A few days later after being constipated, I finally went to the bathroom but because the popcorn had hardened into big clusters in my intestines, it was very painful. About an hour later I started bleeding from the rectum. That was extremely upsetting and scary. Everything always seemed to happen to me on the weekends when I could not reach my doctor. I did not know why I was bleeding. Nobody ever told me not to eat popcorn while taking chemo. I had not associated the popcorn with the bleeding. The bleeding started on a Friday night and continued until Monday afternoon. I was bleeding (what looked like) approximately a teaspoon of blood every half hour and I felt an urge to go to the bathroom every time I would bleed. That feeling alone was terrible. I had been given a magnet with a 24 hour nurse line called Vitaline. At the time, I did not remember that this line also had a physician on-call 24-7. Anyway, I called on Saturday morning to see what I should do. The nurse I spoke with advised me to go to the ER. Before taking her advice, I had presence of mind to ask her two important questions. 1. Was I losing a dangerous amount of blood? And 2. What would they do to me if I went to the ER? She told me I was not in any danger with that amount of bleeding and I could wait until Monday to contact my doctor unless the bleeding got worse. She also let me know that if I went to the ER, I would be examined and scoped. I did not like the sound of that! I decided to wait until Monday. In the meantime, the nurse suggested that the bleeding might be caused by hemorrhoids. I never had hemorrhoids before but she told me they could be caused by the chemo weakening the walls of my intestines. She suggested I try Tucks which might have helped if the bleeding wasn't internal. It turned out that I made the right decision because the bleeding stopped by Monday afternoon. I found out later, after talking to my doctor, that popcorn can have that affect if eaten shortly before or shortly after taking chemo. It was several months before I ate popcorn again!

Keep a Positive Attitude

When we are sick it is easy to sink into depression. It is hard to be happy when you don't feel good. When you are given a cancer diagnosis and know that the road ahead will be a difficult one, it is easy to focus on the pain and anxiety of what lies ahead. Remember to take one step at a time. In the movie, "*What About Bob*" (which is a great movie to watch), the psychiatrist wrote a book called *Baby Steps*. It is a very funny movie but also very true. Don't try to jump ahead and picture a negative outcome. I had heard all kinds of horror stories about chemo which filled me with dread. You have to take one day at a time or baby steps. I had many scary and upsetting things happen but all in all, the chemo was not as bad as I had anticipated. Try to think positive thoughts and plan little things that make you happy. Plan to do something fun after your chemo treatments are finished so you have something to look forward to. Remember that there is new research going on all the time and a new treatment for you may be just around the corner. Doctors and researchers have made so many achievements over the past 40 years. My grandmother had colon cancer 40 years ago and she really suffered with her chemo treatments. Things are so much better today. Keep praying and believe in miracles. They still happen. But for those of you who have difficulty believing in miracles, let me give you something else to consider. When you are given a diagnosis of cancer, your emotions generally reign supreme. Your emotions are fragile because you suddenly realize how vulnerable you are. This fear may play a significant role in your susceptibility to disease and even in your recovery. However, you have a choice in how you feel. You control the way you think and in turn control your emotions which can help or hinder your recovery. The central nervous system and the immune system communicate with each other. Immune cells travel in your blood through your body and come in contact with every other cell. If the immune cells recognize other cells, they leave them alone. But if they do not recognize certain cells, they attack them. Therefore, if the immune cell comes into contact with a cancer cell, it will attack it unless it misidentifies it. The field that studies the correlation between the immune system and the central nervous system is called psychoneuroimmunology. Research has found that the chemical messengers that function broadly in the brain and immune system are the chemical messengers that are most dense in the neural regions that control emotion. They have actually identified a contact point where nerve cells release neurotransmitters which regulate immune cells. What all of this is saying is that your emotions directly relate to your immune system. Therefore, when you are extremely anxious or depressed it can compromise your immune function to the point that it can speed the metastasis of cancer. That information should open your eyes to the reality that your mental attitude plays a part in your recovery.

Join Existing Cancer/Chemo Support Groups in Your Area

Some of your best support may come from being involved in a cancer support group. You will meet other men and women who are going through some of the same things you are going through. They will have a lot of important information they can share with you and maybe you will be able to help one of them. Someone in that group may be able to answer some of your questions that even the doctors or nurses may not be able to answer due to first hand experience. They might think to tell you something helpful that the doctor or nurses might forget such as "don't eat popcorn." It is also good for your spirit to talk to people who are going through the same thing you are so you do not feel so alone. And you may make a friend who will be there for you on a weekend when you may not be able to reach your doctor with a question. I tend to want to be alone when I don't feel well. I just want to stay in bed and isolate myself until I am better. That may be okay when you have the flu but when you have cancer, it is better to connect with a support group. Knowledge is power and support groups provide first hand knowledge. And remember that you can join a group just by talking on the phone if you don't feel like attending a meeting or live too far away. In addition, studies have shown that social isolation doubles the chances of sickness.

Cut Your Hair Before You Lose It

I had long blond hair and hated to cut it so I just let it fall out. This was a mistake because my hair was everywhere. I had to pick it off of my clothes constantly and it filled the vacuum when I would sweep. I was not as upset as most women about losing my hair. My main concern was that I did not want to be sick. I was sick to my stomach for 6 weeks before I was diagnosed with ovarian cancer. Since I had been sick for so long, I was not as concerned with how I looked. I was more concerned about being well and not having a stomach ache or being nauseated. However, I did have one time when I looked in the mirror and began to cry. My hair was falling out by the strands. It was Thanksgiving and my family was gathering at my brother's house just down the street from where we live. I was going to attend too but when I looked in the mirror, I suddenly felt very depressed and decided not to attend. I think I might not have felt so bad if I had gotten my hair cut. It would have given me a little control over the situation.

Wash Your Head Even When You Don't Have Hair

I have always had a sensitive scalp but my scalp became extremely tender when I was taking chemo treatments. It seemed to be especially tender when I was losing my hair. It hurt to even lay my head on my pillow. Buy a mild shampoo or even a baby shampoo and wash your scalp with it when you shower. It made my scalp feel better.

Get a Good Wig and Some Hats or Baseball Caps

A lot of heat escapes from your head especially when you don't have any hair. I started losing my hair in November and even though we live in the south, it was turning cold outside. My scalp was very tender when I was actually losing my hair so I preferred to wear stocking caps around the house. They kept my head warm and were soft on my scalp. I bought a wig at a local wig shop for around $30. It is nice enough but it made my head hot and itchy. They make special wigs with gel on the inside that are much cooler to wear. You cannot always find them in wig shops but most wig catalogs carry them. I bought one from a Paula Young catalog made with "Coolmax Fabric" which they advertise to provide "soothing, itch-free wear and maximum breathability." If you invest in this type of wig you will most likely feel more comfortable. Since I had just moved to a new town, nobody knew me except my family so most of the time I just wore a lot of different baseball caps when I went out. As I mentioned earlier, I did not have a job so I did not need to dress up. It is also good to know that some health insurance policies cover the cost of a wig if your loss of hair is due to chemo treatments. In addition, your wig is a tax deductible expense.

If Your Port Becomes Infected, Have It Removed Right Away

One of the worst experiences for me was getting a port, also known as a vascular access device. Now I believe that a port can be a great help for people who need chemo treatments. When you take chemo, it makes your veins shrink and hide. This makes it difficult for the nurses to find a vein when they need to insert an IV. I had been sick for 6 weeks previous to my diagnosis and then I had surgery. My body was dehydrated which made it even more difficult to find my veins. Nobody explained anything to me about a port before I went in for my first chemo treatment. I had envisioned sitting in a chair with an IV in my arm (at the elbow) receiving the chemo. That is not usually how it is done. If you only need a couple of chemo treatments, they may not suggest a port but most people need more treatments than that so in many cases a port is used. If they give you an IV directly in your arm and do not use a port, they will try to find a vein near your wrist or in your hand. The nurses do not use the crook of your arm near the elbow because they do not want the needle breaking off or coming out if you bend your arm. My doctor ordered 6 chemo treatments of Paclitaxel® and Carboplatin® (one treatment a month for six months). My treatments were an all-day affair. I would go in around 8:30 in the morning and have blood drawn and have an IV inserted (for the times I did not have the port). Then I would see my doctor for a quick exam and answer a few questions regarding how I was feeling and if I was having any side effects from the chemo. Also during this time, I was attended to by one of Dr. Powell's nurses. All of his nurses are kind and empathetic. One nurse in particular (Melinda) was always upbeat and helpful. She continually let me know how much she cared by her kind words and encouragement. After my exam with Dr. Powell, I would go to the chemo room where I would wait until the results of my blood work came back from the lab. Once they had the results, they would hook me up to the IV and I would sit for approximately 6 hours before it was finished. The nurses had a very difficult time finding my veins. The first time I went in for chemo, the nurse searched my lower arms, wrists and hands but all my veins were hiding. She finally found a vein in the back of my hand but stuck me several times before she struck oil! This nurse was careful and compassionate. She did her best to make me comfortable but my hands are very sensitive. So I received my first chemo treatment in my right hand. The chemo nurses were very kind and helpful. They suggested that I get a port because it would be a one time procedure to insert the port and then it would eliminate the need to find a vein every time I came in to get a treatment. Now the thought of having a port inserted under my skin really disgusted me. I had seen a lady with a port protruding out of her chest (near her neck) and it looked awful. It looked alien. However, everyone assured me that it was no big deal and I would be much happier after I had the port. This is like the kiss of death on the soap operas when they say, "nothing will ever separate us" and you know it won't be long until the couple is divorced. I agreed to get the port but I was still apprehensive. It is not as simple a procedure as they lead you to believe. The whole thing takes several hours. You generally have a choice to get the port in your chest or your arm. The port is a catheter which is surgically inserted into a tube that is pulled from a vein in your arm (or chest) through to a larger vein in your chest which leads to your heart. The larger the vein that is used, the less chance that it will be destroyed by the chemo. Also, the larger veins carry the blood faster. The port is approximately the size of a half dollar. The middle of the port is rubbery and can be punctured with a needle that is specially designed to connect with the IV tubing. The port can then be used for blood tests, IV's and even medications so you don't have to be continually stuck with needles. You are prepped for the surgical procedure and an IV is inserted for the anesthesia. Some of my anxiety was due to the fact that my veins were hiding and once again it was difficult for the nurse to find a vein to insert the IV. I admit that I am a big baby when it comes to needles so keep in mind that you will probably have a much better experience if you keep a positive attitude. You are not put out completely but you feel no pain. A local anesthetic is generally used. The procedure is usually performed in radiology where they can use a type of x-ray machine to see what they are doing when they insert and thread the tube. The actual procedure takes about half an hour. I remember the radiologist talking to me while he did the procedure but I kept my eyes shut. My problem began shortly after that. When they had finished the procedure, the nurse applied a type of glue that helps hold the skin together. The problem was that the nurse did not wait for the glue to dry before he put the bandages on. The bandage adhered to my skin so after several days when I was supposed to take off the bandage, part of it would not come off. I called the radiologist and asked what I should do about the bandage and I was told to leave it on and eventually it would fall off. That is what I did, however, I think this is when the area became infected. The bandage eventually did fall off, but a day later the area on my arm around the port became red and began to hurt. Once again, this happened on a weekend when it would have been difficult to reach my doctor. I developed a fever and I was warned not to mess around if the wound became infected since the port led to my heart. I was also under the impression that they may not be able to give me the rest of my chemo treatments if I did not use a port. So I was very upset and concerned. It was a Saturday so I went to the local ER (not New Hanover where I was receiving my regular care since that was 1 ½ hours away). The doctor in the ER had never worked with ports so he did not know what to do. He ended up calling another doctor who said I should be put back on antibiotics. However, he scared me because he said I might have to have the port removed due to the infection. This was upsetting because at that time I thought that there weren't any other options for getting the chemo and I would not be able to receive the rest of my chemo treatments. But that was not the case. When you first get the port, they put you on antibiotics for a week while you heal. Three days after I finished taking the first round of antibiotics is when my port became infected. Four days after taking the second round of antibiotics, I started feeling better and my arm started to look better. But there was a small area in my arm that would not heal. There was a small hole where the port was inserted that just would not close. Two weeks after receiving the port, I went back to the radiologist so he could look at my arm to see why it was not healing. He said it looked pretty good and to just give it more time to heal. All this time I was told to not get the area wet and not let the area rub against anything. The port was inserted on the inside of my left arm. That meant that I had to hold my arm out away from my body all the time. I was supposed to let the air get to it so I did not have it bandaged. I had to sleep in one position with my arm on a pillow and try not to move it all night long. I had to take sponge baths instead of showers so I did not get it wet. And it was winter time and I could not wear a sleeve on that arm. This went on for 2 ½ months! My back ached from having to hold my arm out away from my body and I was cold all the time because I could not wear anything on that arm. I got to use the port twice before it became infected again and I had to have it removed. After they removed the port, I had to return to the hospital four times to have the area cleaned and bandaged due to the infection. I was able to receive my last three chemo treatments in a vein in my hand. I went through all of that pain and aggravation for 2 ½ months only to be able to use the port twice! Some people opt to get another port inserted if the first one becomes infected. I was given that option but did not want to take the chance that the second port might become infected. Besides I only had 3 chemo treatments left. Maybe if I had complained more to my doctor things might have been different but I did not want to be a complainer and did not think that there might be another option. Sometimes we need to be our own advocate and speak up. Doctors cannot read our minds and may not realize what we are experiencing unless we tell them.

A Good Diet Is Important to Your Recovery

When I went in for my first chemo treatment, I was bombarded with information from the nurses and other people who were helping in the chemotherapy room. One benefit that the Zimmer Center offered was the consultation services of a dietician. A good dietician can provide you with important information about what type of diet is best for you and may be able to answer questions for you throughout the duration of your chemo treatments. A balanced diet can also help with side effects such as fatigue. It was suggested to me that I limit the amount of caffeine I drink and make sure I was eating plenty of protein.

Don't Eat Fresh Fruits or Vegetables over the Duration of Your Chemo Treatments

Chemo lowers your immune system and makes you more susceptible to food-borne illnesses. I was tempted to eat salads but I resisted the temptation because I did not want to take the chance of getting sick. You can substitute things for fresh fruit like eating apple sauce instead of apples or eating canned pineapple, peaches, etc. You can eat fresh vegetables as long as you cook them. I love steamed broccoli and cauliflower and they even have cancer fighting agents in them. Thaw meat in the refrigerator and not on the kitchen counter. Cook meat and eggs thoroughly. Avoid raw shellfish and use only pasteurized or processed ciders and juices and pasteurized milk and cheese.

Don't Eat at Fast Food Restaurants or Buffets

For the same reason as not eating fresh fruits or vegetables, you should not eat fast foods or eat at buffets. There is a greater risk of contacting E-Coli in those situations and when you are taking chemo, your immune system is compromised. It is a good idea to stay away from fast food restaurants anyway. This should be a time when you start eating healthier if you have not been eating that way before.

Go on a Soft Food or Liquid Diet a Few Days Before and After Each Chemo Treatment

This goes along with not eating popcorn. I learned that I felt much better if I only ate soft food or liquids like soup a few days before and after each chemo treatment. The chemo made everything I ate harden up during digestion. I would have a couple of days of constipation and feeling like I had to use the bathroom. Although it was uncomfortable, I never had any bleeding except for the time that I ate popcorn. I just felt a lot better when I only ate soup or pudding or soft foods during those few days. It took me a while to learn this so I hope this will help you.

Use a Stool Softener

For the same reasons I mentioned above, you may want to use a stool softener. I recommend Senokot because it did not cause bloating or gas and it is a natural vegetable laxative. I did not need it every month but definitely used it after eating the popcorn! I suggest taking 2 pills once a day for however many days you feel you need it but follow the directions on the bottle. One of the chemo nurses said some people take as many as 4 a day. Chemo treatments can actually cause constipation in some people and sometimes the medications you take to reduce the side effects of the chemo can cause constipation. It is important to drink plenty of fluids to keep your stool soft. The usual recommendation is at least eight 8-ounce glasses per day. Increasing the fiber in your diet can also help but be sure to check with your doctor first because a high fiber diet is not recommended for certain types of cancer. Exercise can also help keep you regulated.

If You Have to Get a Shot to Increase Your White Blood Cell Count, Take Claritin® to Help with the Aching

I had to get a shot (Neulasta®) each month a day after receiving the chemo to increase my white blood cell count. Chemo tends to decrease your white blood cell count so it is not uncommon to need this shot. I was also told by one of the chemo nurses that taking antibiotics may decrease your white blood cell count. I had taken several rounds of antibiotics during this whole ordeal. Anyway, the shot has a side affect which is that it makes the bones in your legs ache. It also made my back and feet ache terribly. I tried soaking my feet in warm water and rubbing my feet and legs but nothing helped. The only thing that helped was taking Claritin®. The chemo nurses said that a study was being done at Duke University regarding how Claritin® helps the aching after taking Neulasta® to increase the white blood cells and that they (the nurses) recommend taking it to their patients. It really helped. Start taking it the evening that you get the shot (before you start to ache) and take one a day for the next several days until the aching stops. With me, the aching usually started 1 to 2 days after I received the shot and the aching lasted 3 to 4 days. I tried other things but Claritin® was the best.

Try to Stay off of Your Feet as Much as Possible After Getting the Neulasta® Shot

Another thing that helps with the aching is to try to stay off of your feet as much as possible. I made the mistake of taking a long walk a day after getting the shot since it was recommended that I get some exercise. However, this made the aching worse. I found that I felt the best if I just laid in bed and took Claritin® for a few days. This is not to say that you should stay in bed all of the time. Do what feels best for you but it may help to plan your exercise around the time when any side effects from Neulasta® have passed.

Drink a Lot of Water Prior to Getting Any Blood Tests or Chemo Treatments If You Do Not Have a Port

As I mentioned earlier, when you receive chemo, it makes your veins shrink and hide making it difficult for the nurses to find a vein to draw blood or administer the chemo. Water helps to plump up the veins so drink a lot of water before you go in for any blood work. Drinking eight 8-ounce glasses of water a day is a good thing anyway. This is just another reason to drink a lot of water.

Eat Protein to Help with Your White Blood Cell Count

I had a low white blood cell count even before my first chemo treatment. It had never been a problem before but something made it low at the time I was diagnosed with ovarian cancer. I was sick for 6 weeks prior to my diagnosis and I was not eating much so this may have attributed to the low count. I was also told by a nurse that sometimes taking antibiotics can lower the white blood cell count. I had taken antibiotics when I was sick because the doctor at the Urgent Care Center where I went said that I could have a parasite and that could be what was causing my illness. So he prescribed an antibiotic right away while we waited for the results of the blood test. As you know, it turned out not to be parasites. Besides already having a low white blood cell count, chemo lowers the white blood cell count. So I was a candidate for receiving a shot to increase my white blood cells. In fact, they would not give me the chemo unless I received the shot because your white blood cell count has to be in a certain range before they will give you chemo. I researched the internet and asked both my doctor and several nurses what I could do to increase my white blood cell count. The only thing I could find besides taking a pill or a shot, was to eat protein. A normal white blood cell count range is from 4.6 to 10.2. My count started at 4.7 and went as low as 2.2.

Antibiotics Seem to Decrease the White Blood Cell Count

As I mentioned earlier, antibiotics seem to decrease the white blood cell count. Several chemo nurses suggested this and it proved true for me. I kept track of my white blood cell count each month when they drew blood for my cbc. I made a chart on my computer at home and also recorded every time I took antibiotics. I took antibiotics 5 separate times while I was sick and while taking chemo. I noticed that each time I took the antibiotics, my white blood cell count was lower than the times I was not taking antibiotics.

Chemotherapy Can Cause Anemia

Anemia is the result of the bone marrow's inability to produce red blood cells. Red blood cells carry oxygen to every area of your body. If there are not enough red blood cells then your body will not get enough oxygen to operate efficiently. Anemia can cause several symptoms or problems in and of itself. You may feel fatigued (weak, tired and sleepy), feel like your heart is pounding and beating very fast, have shortness of breath, or feel dizzy or faint. There is a shot to stimulate your bone marrow to increase the production of red blood cells just like the shot to increase white blood cells. My problem was insufficient white blood cells. Along with getting the shot, you should have well-balanced meals, get plenty of sleep and don't try to do everything yourself. Learn to rest and accept help from friends and family.

Chemotherapy Can Cause Blood Clotting Problems

Along with the bone marrow's inability to produce white and red blood cells, chemo can also cause the bone marrow to stop or slow down the production of platelets. Platelets are the blood cells that help stop any bleeding by making blood clots. If you do not have enough platelets, you will bleed and or bruise more easily. If your bone marrow is not producing enough platelets, you may have symptoms such as pin-point red dots under your skin, bruising, nose bleeds, gums bleeding, vaginal bleeding, headaches, dark or bloody stool, pinkish colored urine, and blurred or changes in your vision. Blood work is always taken before administering chemotherapy and a complete blood count is included in that blood work. If your platelets are low, your doctor may offer medicine to stimulate your bone marrow to produce more platelets or he may suggest a platelet transfusion.

Take a Lot of Showers or Baths

This sounds like common sense but when you are taking chemo, you lose your energy and it is easy to stay in your pajamas or just throw on some old clothes. Sometimes you have to push yourself to get moving or even to take a shower. But after you take a shower or a bath, you always feel better. There is something refreshing about feeling clean and smelling good. It is also nice to feel the sensation of the warm water. In addition, taking a hot bath or shower can help you relax and sleep better.

Watch a Lot of Comedies

I'm a true believer that laughter is the best medicine. My brother & sister-in-law bought me a portable dvd player with headphones which I took with me each time I went for a chemo treatment. It was a good distraction while I sat there for 6 hours. I watched funny movies and some old time sitcoms which I bought ahead of time. One movie I highly recommend is *Evan Almighty* starring Steve Carell. It is not only funny but has a great message (i.e. "have faith"). The sitcoms I bought were nice because they were old ones from when I was a kid and they brought back good memories as I watched them. I was probably the only one in the chemo room who was laughing while I was receiving chemo. It really is good to take your mind off of your troubles and just try to relax. My friends and family bought me funny movies that I could watch at home while I was recuperating. It gave us something to do together and kept us laughing instead of focusing on my condition.

Some Depression Is Normal

Chemo zaps the body of energy and when you are fatigued, depression is soon to follow. If you have been given a less than perfect prognosis, if you are undergoing months of chemotherapy or radiation, if you are feeling sick or hate the way you look when you look in the mirror due to hair loss, bloating or some other side effect, it is easy to become depressed. The most important thing to do is to not give up hope. Believe in a positive outcome and believe in yourself. Decide that you are going to do everything possible to beat the cancer. It is also important for you to talk about your feelings. This may be the most fearful and anxiety ridden time of your life. It is great to have a friend or family member to talk to but it is even better to be able to talk to a nurse, a therapist or another cancer patient or cancer survivor. That is one reason why it is helpful to join existing cancer/chemo support groups in your area. Eating a good diet, exercising and getting enough rest are also important for good mental health. Try to stay away from stressful situations as much as possible. Stress is one of the worst things to have in your life, especially now. Think of little things that make you happy and surround yourself with as many of them as you can. Sometimes just having flowers in your room can change your mood.

Read positive and uplifting books and watch a lot of comedies. Think of ways you can help someone else. Listen to your favorite music. Don't focus on the negatives. Keep believing in miracles and keep praying. God is listening. If you do not understand something about your treatment or recovery, write down your questions and ask your doctor at your next appointment. Empower yourself with knowledge.

Keep Track of When You Feel Poorly After Each Chemo Treatment So You Know What to Expect Each Time

My first chemo treatment was the worst. I guess I should rephrase that. The side affects after my first chemo treatment were the worst. Three days after my first treatment, I was standing in the kitchen when I began to feel sick. I felt nauseated and also like I was going to have diarrhea. At the same time, my whole body started to severely tingle almost like I was being zapped by a stun gun. I broke out in a cold sweat and my ears went shut (like when you are flying at a high altitude). It was a terrible experience. However, my doctor had prescribed a pill (Prochlorperazine®) that was supposed to help if I became nauseated so I took it right away when I started feeling sick. I was already taking other pills for the nausea but this pill turned off nausea responses in the brain while the other nausea pills worked in the stomach. I felt terrible for about half an hour and then the pill must have kicked in because I started feeling better. I kept track of when I felt bad on a calendar so I could see if there was a pattern of how I felt each month. That way I could be prepared. I asked my doctor if I could take that pill even if I did not feel bad. In other words, I planned to take the pill on the third day after the chemo treatment each month before I had any reaction to the chemo. As *Barney Fife* would say "Nip it, nip it, nip it." Fortunately, I did not have that experience again and each chemo treatment was a little better than the last one (with the exception of the popcorn incident).

Be Aware That Some Antibiotics Cause Allergic Reactions and Some Reactions (If They Are Severe) Can Cause a Fever

When my port became infected the second time, my local doctor prescribed Septra DS® which is a strong antibiotic. It turns out that I am allergic to it but I did not know that at the time because I had never taken it before. I had been taking it for 8 days when I woke up one morning covered in a red rash and my face was bright red. I was aching and I had a fever of 102. I called a nurse at the hospital where I received my chemo treatments and she said I needed to come in right away. Before I went in, I called my local MD who suggested I might be having an allergic reaction to the antibiotic. He told me to stop taking it right away which I did. I still went in to the Zimmer Center to see the nurse who ordered some blood work. She said she did not believe it was an allergic reaction since I had a fever. As it turned out, it was a severe allergic reaction to the antibiotic. In some cases, a severe allergic reaction can cause a fever. A day after I quit taking it I was fine.

Bad Things Usually Happen on Weekends When You May Not Be Able to Reach Your Doctor. Ask for a 24-Hour Emergency Hotline Where You Can Get Questions Answered That May Help You Decide If You Need to Go to an ER

It was my luck that when something bad happened, it always happened on the weekend when it was difficult to reach my doctor. If you are like me, it is scary when something strange happens to your body. I tend to become alarmed and worry that the situation is worse than it is. One time my port became infected and I had a 102 degree fever. This started on a Friday night. Another time I had rectal bleeding. This also started on a Friday night. These are just two examples. Fortunately, New Hanover Medical Center had provided me with a 24 hour nurse hotline called Vitaline which also provides contact with a physician on-call 24-7. Always be prepared (as much as possible) for things to happen on the weekend. If you are starting to feel bad or starting to have a problem on a Thursday or Friday, don't put off making a phone call to your doctor. Things always seem to get worse on the weekend when you may not be able to reach your doctor. Just call to see if you need to do something before your situation worsens. And remember to ask if there is a 24 hour hotline that you can use.

Accept Help from Your Family and Friends. Don't Try to Do Everything Yourself

I always hate asking for help. I try to be self-sufficient. However, sometimes you need to ask for help. I am single so right off the bat I do not have a significant other to help me. I was fortunate to have my mother who came to my rescue and helped nurse me back to health. But she could not do it all. She was 80 years old and she needed help too. My mother and I had just moved to North Carolina so that we could be near my brother and his family. We bought a house right down the street from his house. Little did I know what a blessing that would be. When I was diagnosed with ovarian cancer, I was referred to a specialist at a hospital 1 ½ hours away in a town I had never been to before. I did not know my way around and I was sick so I was in no condition to be driving anyway. My mother was 80 and I did not want her driving around in an area she did not know either. Thank God that my brother (the Rev. Dr. William G. Waun) was willing and able to take me to my first couple of treatments until I felt well enough to drive myself and had learned the way. He had to take time off from his job and spend the whole day sitting with me while I received the chemo. He also came to my rescue on more than one occasion when I called him at home because something had happened and I needed his moral support. My sister-in-law (Cynthia) researched my condition on the internet and provided me with information and questions that I could ask my doctor when I was too sick to do the research myself. She also made me some meals and went to the store for me. My friends sent flowers, cards and letters. Most of my friends were in other states since I had just moved here. My mother did the most for me. She went to every chemo treatment with me. She made me homemade soups and stews when I didn't want to eat. She ran to the grocery store and bought me whatever I needed or wanted. She sat with me, laughed with me, cried with me and prayed with me. I don't know what I would have done without her. Accept the help and love that others offer. You can pay it back or pay it forward when you feel better.

Keep Track of Your CA-125 Scores

A CA-125 is a blood test which is an indicator for cancer The blood contains substances at certain levels that are called tumor markers. When the tumor markers rise above a specified range, it may indicate cancer. Please note that tumor markers are not an absolute when predicting cancer but they are a great tool for doctors to use. The tests usually used for breast cancer are the CA15-3 or the CA 27-29. The test for ovarian cancer is generally the CA-125. My first CA-125 score was 126. It is supposed to be below 30 (between 4.0 – 30.2). After the surgery it came down to 32.1. After my first chemo treatment my score was 9.4 and after my last chemo treatment my score was 4. The chemo nurses told me that they could not believe how low my score was. They said there are people walking around who have never had cancer and have scores higher than mine. I had a lot of people praying for me and I also followed my doctor's orders. I will continue to go to follow up exams beginning with 3 month intervals where they will monitor my CA-125 score. I have also learned of another blood test called OvaSure (developed by Yale University researchers) that claims to detect early-stage ovarian cancer with 99% accuracy.

Wash Your Hands

When you are taking chemo, your immune system is compromised and you are more susceptible to germs and illness. I was told not to clean or even be around any litter boxes, bird cages or fish tanks. I was also told not to have close contact with other people such as shaking hands or hugging people in church. Most germs are passed by touching someone or something. That is why it is so important to wash your hands a lot. When you are taking chemo, you have little resistance to fight off the germs like you normally would have. I have a parrot and a cat. While I was on chemo, my mother cleaned my bird's cage and cleaned out my cat's litter box. I should write an entire chapter on what a great mother I have. I may have taken things a little further than I had to but I did not go out of the house very much during the 6 months that I was taking chemo. I would sit in my back yard a lot but that was not near any people. I went out a few times to the grocery store and a few clothing stores around Christmas time but I stayed away from people as much as I could. I did not go anywhere where I would be in an enclosed place with people for any period of time. I did not go to church or the movie theater. I did not get in cars with people except for my mother. I asked that friends and family not come over if they were not feeling well and we did not have any company come and stay with us at our house during that time. I felt bad enough with what I was going through without making it worse by getting a cold or the flu which could have turned into something much worse due to a low resistance. I was fortunate in that I did not get a cold or the flu during that time. I also remembered to constantly wash my hands.

Keep Your Distance Around Children. Your Immune System Is Low and Children Spread Germs

I guess this is common sense but it is not always easy to stay away from children. If you are a mother with small children, you will have to ignore this point except that you might want to keep other small children from coming into your home. And you might want to make sure your children wash their hands a lot.

Be Careful Not to Cut Yourself

This applies to manicuring your finger and toe nails, flossing your teeth and shaving along with accidental cuts. Don't pinch or squeeze pimples. Don't get any immunizations while taking chemo. Don't scratch yourself too hard or rub yourself too hard when you are drying off after a shower. Stay away from standing water which can breed germs (i.e., bird baths, humidifiers and public bathroom sinks). Be sure to clean any cuts right away with soap and antiseptics.

Get a Good Hand Cream

Washing your hands all the time tends to make them dry. Buy a good moisturizer for your hands to keep the skin from cracking making you more vulnerable to germs. I found a cream I liked that provided moisture without being greasy. I bought an extra tube to keep in my car.

Keep Vaseline on Hand

Chemo generally dries out the mucus membrane in your body such as the inside of your nose and mouth. I put Vaseline in my nostrils at night to keep them from drying up and bleeding. I am prone to nosebleeds but never had one during the six months that I was taking chemo. As long as I knew the possibility of what to expect or what could happen, I took precautions to prevent it.

Don't Use Mouthwashes That Contain Alcohol

It is important to remember to take care of your teeth when you are on chemo. There were days when I did not feel like doing anything including brushing my teeth. However, I did not want more problems than I already had so I flossed and brushed regularly. The one thing I skipped while on chemo was rinsing with a mouthwash. Most mouthwashes contain alcohol which can really burn your mouth if it is dry from taking chemo. You may want to use a soft toothbrush and rinse your mouth with warm water when your gums are sore. You can also use a mouthwash with sodium bicarbonate (baking soda) which should not irritate your gums.

Chemo Can Make Your Mouth Dry

Drink a lot of water and always carry a bottle of water with you. If you do not have mouth sores, I suggest drinking lemonade. Sweet and tart foods tend to generate saliva. I kept popsicles on hand. I also like to chew gum because it satisfies my sweet tooth but it also helps make saliva. In addition, it is a good idea to use lip balm to keep your lips from becoming dry.

Soft Foods Are Easier on the Mouth and Throat

Mouth sores, tender gums, and a sore throat or esophagus often result from radiation or chemotherapy. If this happens, you should consult with your doctor because it could be due to an unrelated dental problem and your doctor may be able to give you medicine that will help to control mouth and throat pain. Be aware that certain foods may irritate an already tender mouth or make chewing difficult. As I stated earlier, I went on a soft food or liquid diet a few days prior to my chemo treatment and a few days after. I did not have any trouble with mouth or throat sores but the soft diet helped with digestion. On the same note, you will want to avoid citrus fruits such as oranges, grapefruit and lemons, and spicy or salty foods. Here are some soft foods you may want to try:

- Instant mashed potatoes
- Milkshakes
- Applesauce or canned peaches
- Cottage cheese or yogurt
- Macaroni and cheese
- Custards, puddings and gelatin

- Ice cream
- Scrambled eggs
- Oatmeal

Stay Away from Sugar-Free Foods

Sorbitol, which is a sugar substitute that is used in many sugar-free foods, can cause diarrhea. I made the mistake of eating some sugar-free ice cream which caused cramping and diarrhea. Sugar-free gum can do the same thing. This isn't the time to be dieting so ditch the sugar-free foods.

Some Hospitals Provide Financial Help

I had an unusual situation because my job in Georgia had ended and I moved to North Carolina to live near my brother and his family. I had only been in North Carolina for a few weeks when I started to get sick so I had not had time to find a job. I was paying for my own health insurance. I have never gone without health insurance even though I have been very healthy all of my life. The one thing I did change was that I decided to make my annual deduction higher and also selected a plan where the percentage I paid was higher so my monthly payments would be lower. It was like Murphy's Law was just waiting to jump out and hit me in the head! And it did because right after changing my policy, I got sick. When I first became ill I was covered under my Georgia policy for the first month. Then it switched to my North Carolina policy. The problem was that I had to meet my Georgia deductible in November and then meet my North Carolina deductible in December. Then I had to pay another North Carolina deductible in January because it was a new year! Besides all of the deductibles, I had to pay 30% of my medical expenses. 30% may not sound like that much but when you are dealing with hospital stays and shots that cost $7000 each, it really adds up. On top of all of that, I was unemployed so I didn't have any income. One day while I was sitting in the chemo chair, I heard one of the chemo nurses telling another patient about some financial help. When she came over to check on me, I asked her about financial assistance and she told me about a program the hospital has for which I might be eligible. She even went and got me the paperwork. I applied, said a prayer and held my breath for several weeks until I received a letter stating that I had been approved through March. That was wonderful news since March 24th was my final chemo treatment. This particular financial assistance program did not pay for everything associated with the hospital. I still had to pay for each doctor visit and for anything associated with radiology such as getting the port. But my insurance paid for 70% of those things so at least I was not responsible for as much. It was a huge relief to receive this financial help from the hospital since I was not eligible for any government help. So, if you are in need of financial help, it can't hurt to at least ask if your hospital has a financial program.

Corresponding therapies

There are many other types of therapy you can receive while taking chemotherapy which can help you through this difficult time. They can help with the healing of your mind and body while reducing stress and easing side effects. As a licensed professional counselor, I highly recommend counseling therapy. Counseling can include many other therapies such as journaling, art therapy, imagery, rhythmic breathing and visualization. I also suggest the following:

Massage therapy

The Zimmer Center where I received my chemo treatments offered massage therapy during my treatment. Massage therapy uses different styles of touch, stroking and manipulation of the muscles to help you relax and release tension.

Pet therapy

The Zimmer Center also offered pet therapy. During chemo treatments a pet therapist would come for a visit with a dog. This is an animal that has been trained to work with sick or injured people. The pet therapist would walk the dog around the chemo room and ask patients if they would like to pet or talk to the dog. Animals are generally accepting of anyone. They do not judge us by our looks or loss of hair. It is comforting to touch a dog or cat and have them relate to you. It has even been proven that stroking a cat or dog can decrease your blood pressure.

Biofeedback

Biofeedback teaches you how to control different body functions such as blood pressure, heart rate, breathing, and muscle tension that normally were considered involuntarily. This is usually done with the use of a machine where you can learn by watching monitoring instruments attached to your body that record changes in your physiology. Then, eventually, you will have a better self-regulation without the aid of those devices. There are also other means of reading biofeedback such as a chemically coated card which detects rises and falls in your skin temperature or hormonal changes. Biofeedback is a good tool to help you when you are tense and anxious and need to learn how to relax.

Progressive relaxation

This is a method where you sit in a comfortable chair or lay down in a quiet atmosphere. You slowly take a deep breath and concentrate on the muscles in your feet. Contract and relax those muscles and then exhale. You continue to breath while contracting and relaxing muscles in your legs and on up in your body finishing with the muscles in your face. Each time you exhale and release your muscles, you release tension and relax that part of your body.

Visualization

I mentioned visualization earlier but want to touch on it again because many people use it to fight cancerous tumors. By using visualization, you can picture the tumor in your mind and think of the chemotherapy as soldiers or bombs crashing into the tumor to destroy it. You can create whatever picture you want to use and picture it often throughout the day as you think about eliminating the cancer.

Reframing and Thought Stopping

Reframing is changing the way you talk to yourself. It is a conscious change of an automatic thought from something negative or unrealistic to something positive, neutral, or objective. Thought stopping is interrupting your thoughts by ordering them to stop. When you feel anxious or upset, this is a sign that your thoughts are making you feel that way. If you have a belief about something such as, "I know I will get sick whenever I have a chemo treatment," this is jumping to a conclusion. You may not get sick every time you have a chemo treatment and in fact, you may not get sick at all. But when you have these kinds of thoughts, they add to your anxiety and stress. The way to change those thoughts and consequential feelings is to use thought stopping. You can combine your thought stopping with reframing to improve the way you feel. In other words, when you are anxious or worried about something, your body will usually cue you by making your heart beat faster or you will get sweaty palms. When you have these types of cues, think about what is going on in your head. If you are having negative or unrealistic thoughts or jumping to conclusions, then tell yourself to stop. Realize what you are doing to yourself. Then use reframing to replace that negative thought with one that is more realistic or objective.

Hypnosis

The use of hypnosis can help to reduce pain and anxiety. Hypnosis places you in a deep relaxed state of mind. A qualified hypnotist may be able to help you with many side effects.

Prayer and meditation

For me, prayer was a given. The first thing I did when I received my diagnosis was to pray. I know God is in control of my life and I cried out to Him for His help. Every time I was scared or uncertain, I prayed. When I felt alone, I prayed. I continue to pray and listen for His answers. I am fortunate in that I have many Christian friends and family members who prayed with me and for me. My brother who is a minister and chaplain in the Navy anointed me with oil and prayed for my healing. Don't underestimate the power of prayer. Along with prayer there is meditation. Meditation is a form of relaxing and being quiet or listening. By being quiet and focusing on something specific such as killing the cancer cells or listening for an answer from God, you are freeing your mind from distractions and releasing stress from your body.

My prayer for you is that you will use this time in your life to stop any negative behavior and replace it with a renewed spirit. I hope that you will read this book and use it as you go through your own journey and that it will help you along the way. I believe that God wanted me to stop and pay attention to Him. I usually have to learn things the hard way in life but once I learn a lesson, I remember it. God is opening my eyes to the pain and hardships of others. Now it is my turn to do what I can for other people who are going through difficult times and while easing their pain, help them to see that God is there for them too.

Ovarian Cancer Info

The following information was taken from The American Cancer Society website and the cancer-info-guide.com website:

Ovarian cancer is one of the most common types of cancers in women. According to the research studies, ovarian cancer ranks fifth in cancer deaths among women. The chances of surviving ovarian cancer are better if the cancer is found early. But because the disease is difficult to detect in its early stage, only about 20% of ovarian cancers are found before tumor growth has spread into adjacent tissues and organs beyond the ovaries.

Stages:

Stage I: The cancer is still contained within the ovary (or ovaries).

Stage 1A: Cancer has developed in one ovary and the tumor is confined to the inside of the ovary. There is no cancer on the outer surface of the ovary. Laboratory examination of washings from the abdomen and pelvis did not find any cancer cells.

Stage 1B: Cancer has developed within both ovaries without any tumor on their outer surfaces. Laboratory examination of washings from the abdomen and pelvis did not find any cancer cells.

Stage 1C: The cancer is present in one or both ovaries and 1 or more of the following are present:

Cancer on the outer surface of at least one of the ovaries

In the case of cystic tumors (fluid-filled tumors), the capsule (outer wall of the tumor) has ruptured.

Laboratory examination found cancer cells in fluid or washings from the abdomen.

Stage II: The cancer is in one or both ovaries and has involved other organs (such as the uterus, fallopian tubes, bladder, the sigmoid colon, or the rectum) within the pelvis.

Stage IIA: The cancer has spread to or has actually invaded the uterus or the fallopian tubes, or both. Laboratory examination of washings from the abdomen did not find any cancer cells.

Stage IIB: The cancer has spread to other nearby pelvic organs such as the bladder, the sigmoid colon, or the rectum. Laboratory examination of washings from the abdomen did not find any cancer cells.

Stage IIC: The cancer has spread to pelvic organs as in stages IIA or IIB and laboratory examination of washings from the abdomen found evidence of cancer cells.

Stage III: The cancer involves 1 or both ovaries, and 1 or both of the following are present: (1) cancer has spread beyond the pelvis to the lining of the abdomen; (2) cancer has spread to lymph nodes.

Stage IIIA: During the staging operation, the surgeon can see cancer involving the ovary or ovaries, but no cancer is grossly visible (can be seen without using a microscope) in the abdomen and the cancer has not spread to lymph nodes. However, when biopsies are checked under a microscope, tiny deposits of cancer are found in the lining of the upper abdomen.

Stage IIIB: There is cancer in one or both ovaries, and deposits of cancer large enough for the surgeon to see, but smaller than 2 cm across, are present in the abdomen. Cancer has not spread to the lymph nodes.

Stage IIIC: The cancer is in one or both ovaries, and one or both of the following are present:

Cancer has spread to lymph nodes.

Deposits of cancer larger than 2 cm across are seen in the abdomen.

Stage IV: This is the most advanced stage of ovarian cancer. The cancer is in one or both ovaries. Distant metastasis (spread of the cancer to the inside of the liver, the lungs, or other organs located outside of the peritoneal cavity) has occurred. Finding ovarian cancer cells in pleural fluid (from the cavity that surrounds the lungs) is also evidence of stage IV disease.

Symptoms:

Ovarian cancer symptoms are nonspecific and mimic those of many other more common conditions, including digestive and bladder disorders. It isn't unusual for a woman with ovarian cancer to be diagnosed with another condition before finally learning she has cancer. The key seems to be persistent or worsening signs and symptoms. With most digestive disorders, symptoms tend to come and go, or they occur in certain situations or after eating certain foods. With ovarian cancer, there's typically little fluctuation where the symptoms are constant and gradually worsen. The most common symptoms are pain or swelling in the belly and gas. Other symptoms are diarrhea or constipation, or an upset stomach. Symptoms may include:

- Pressure or pain in the abdomen, pelvis, back or legs.
- A swollen or bloated abdomen
- Nausea, indigestion, gas, constipation, or diarrhea.

- Feeling very tired all the time.
- Shortness of breath.
- Feeling the need to urinate often.
- Unusual vaginal bleeding (heavy periods, or bleeding after menopause).

Resources

Ovarian Cancer Staging Information taken from:
http://www.cancer.org/docroot/CRI/content/CRI_2_4_3X_How_is_ovarian_cancer_staged_33.asp?sitearea=CRI

Ovarian Cancer Symptom Information taken from:
http://www.cancer-info-guide.com/ovarian-cancer.html

Other Resource used:
U.S. Dept of Health and Human Services (1999), Chemotherapy and You, NIH Publication

Author's Note

No financial gain was received by the author from the Zimmer Center, New Hanover Regional Medical Center or any other company associated with any brand name mentioned. This publication is designed to provide accurate and authoritative information in regard to the subject matter covered. It is sold with the understanding that the author is not engaged in rendering psychological, financial, legal, or other professional services. If expert assistance or counseling is needed, the services of a competent professional should be sought.

CPSIA information can be obtained at www.ICGtesting.com
Printed in the USA
BVOW05s0156110814

362360BV00001B/145/P

9 781608 130894